Diabetes is a Bully!

Pumps are Snitches, but we must PUSH THROUGH

Carmella J Bell, MS, LMFT-A

Table of Contents

I dedicate this book to my brother, Andre, who believed in me, challenged me and held me accountable for getting this book out into the world. I love you more than you will ever know, no matter what.

I also dedicate this book to my late Aunt Carolyn. She taught me so much. She was strong, willing and determined. If it were not for her, I may never have thought I could help other people with diabetes.

Lastly, I dedicate this book to my son Devin who is the ultimate hero! You amaze me with how you manage this condition day to day. Your strength and resilience is a blessing from God. You helped me to understand how involved a diabetes diagnosis can be.

Ultimately, you taught me that I need to share what I have learned with all people with diabetes.

Introduction

Maybe you picked up this book, or somebody gave it to you. There is a good possibility that it took every effort for you to open it up because you are overwhelmed. You do not want to talk any more about the diagnosis you have received, but it is there. It is real.

Everyday highs and lows, no matter what the number says, you have been diagnosed with diabetes. Currently, there is no cure. Despite that, I am here to tell you that you can live a full, healthy, happy life.

People with type 2 diabetes deserve a better standard of care, better than the one currently being administered. It's time to stop accepting the diabetes status quo and start fighting for your life.

There are times when it is so overwhelming that all you want to do is give up. But I hope that in this book, I can provide you with encouragement, hope, and some practical skills that you can use to push through.

Choose life. Live long and healthy!

CHAPTER ONE

This Book May Not Be for You

This book is not for everyone. You don't know how hard it has been to get used to that idea. I want to help everyone. I want to see everyone succeed at kicking diabetes in the butt, but I had to come to terms with the truth. I cannot help everyone, and I was not meant to. There is a group of people whom I understand, and they understand me. We deal with the same things every day. We don't have to preface everything we say. We are not negative. Sometimes we are tired. Sometimes we don't want to play by the rules of diabetes. Sometimes we just want to skip checking glucose levels, forget taking shots, eat what we want or let our kids eat what they want. We want all of this and for the pancreas to do its job. You know, like everyone else!

The reality for most is this is not our reality. I am tired of "Polly Positive" subtly putting me down when I am having a rough day. I might be feeling beat up because I didn't get my son's doses right. Polly sympathizes, but she wants me to perk up. I will eventually, but right now I am a little bummed. I want to get it right. I want him to feel good all the time. I want to know what I am doing is going to keep him healthy and alive for years to come. I know there is no perfection in this process, but I want to get it right! Since I didn't, I want to be one with my feelings. One with my reality. One with the ups and downs of managing diabetes.

With that said, this book is for people with Type 2 Diabetes who have been struggling to manage their condition. By struggling, I mean, aside from knowing you need to watch your sugar, there isn't much you could tell me about diabetes. You might know what it is, but you don't know how to manage it. Most days you eat what you want when you want. You acknowledge with much conviction that, "I only test x amount of times a day/week and that how it is going to be." You only administer insulin when you feel you need it (i.e. when your vision gets blurry, you are urinating like a faucet, you have headaches, etc.).

If I were to ask you about scales, measuring cups, labels and serving sizes, you would scrunch your forehead and look confused. You are thinking, "Measure for what?" You eat out often, maybe several times a week or even several times a day. The truth is, we cannot control what other people put in our food. Many people struggling with diabetes don't count carbs. Some of you may feel resentful, angry, and or that your body has betrayed you. You rebel against anything you are supposed to do because you are upset with how unrecognizable your life has become. For all these reasons and more, we are on course for the perfect storm. That storm is going to land you in an emergency room, with your family in the waiting room wondering if you are going to make it. They would be wondering if you are going to be in a diabetic coma if you had a stroke or a heart attack. They will be wondering if you are going to live or die.

Ouch! Did that hurt? A little uncomfortable? I hope it didn't feel judgmental because that is not my intention. I wrote this book for you!

I was inducted into the diabetes life by way of my son's failed pancreas in November 2012. I know first-hand how hard it is to deal with this condition every day. I have watched people close to me manage and mismanage their diabetes for years. However, it wasn't until diabetes crashed our party that I was forced to learn quickly, not only what it meant to have diabetes, but what it takes to survive.

Like many people, I thought that people with diabetes are educated about their condition (some are). They know what they should and should not eat (some do). I thought people with diabetes knew how to follow through with testing their blood and taking insulin as directed. I thought dialysis, heart attacks, strokes, loss of eyesight and amputations were eventually going to happen to all people with diabetes. What did I know? Nothing.

My aunt, Lord rest her soul, was a long time suffer from diabetes. I knew my aunt needed to eat better, but I didn't know exactly what she was supposed to be doing. Looking back on her life, no real help was ever offered to her. There were only high-level conversations with her doctors, judgment from relatives, and shame for not knowing how to take care of herself.

After my son's diagnosis, I started meeting more and more people with type 2 diabetes. At that point, I thought type 2 was the same as type 1. After many conversations and a lot of reading, I learned this was not the case. So, I made it my mission to talk to people dealing with type 2 to find out more about the type 2 experience.

More surprisingly, I discovered there are a lot of people with diabetes who don't understand their diagnosis. They don't know how to eat better without feeling deprived. They receive a lot of criticism from family and friends who think they know what is best. They go to doctors who do not practice from a holistic perspective. These doctors don't have time to dig as deep as they'd like, so they just adjust the medication and send patients on their way.

I didn't know what I was witnessing as I watched my aunt eat cake, ice cream, and cookies at family parties. This behavior is not preferred, but it also is not detrimental. In a perfect world, we would all swap our carb loaded breakfasts for veggie smoothies, exercise 7 days a week, and meditate for an hour a day. No one would be overweight, we would never lose our tempers, and we would sing Kumbaya all day. This is the real world, so this is never going to happen.

As she ate her cake and cookies, not once did my aunt test her blood or attempt to take any insulin to cover those sweet treats. I didn't know that I was idly sitting by while my aunt played Russian Roulette with her life by the way she mismanaged her diabetes.

What I know for sure, when you know better, you do better. It will not happen again. Not on my watch.

My realization didn't come until after my son was diagnosed and we were thrust into the bottles (the ones with the little orange caps). It was volatile. His blood sugars were up and down, and we were going crazy in between. We later switched to insulin pens which were more convenient, but he grew tired of shots. Then, we switched to a pump. The pump has been a tremendous benefit in helping us fine tune our practices and meal plans to keep his glucose levels on track. We still struggle with overnight highs, but things are looking up.

After my son's diagnosis and my crash course in Diabetes 101, I learned that my aunt's diabetes regimen was like my son's. They were even on the same medication. I crunched the numbers, reveling in the similarities. It felt good to know a warrior in the struggle. Someone who knew this process was not about perfection. I know that, no matter how hard I try, something can always throw me off my game. Just before I started doing my happy dance, I realized one thing. She was doing it all wrong! Very wrong. This behavior needed to stop immediately.

My aunt had been living with diabetes for 25 or more years. She had grown accustomed to her casual management style, and routine hospital stays. My aunt thought she knew everything already, and so she was choosing to do it her way. In a way, I am thankful for diabetes because diabetes is what allowed me to grow closer to my aunt and cherish the time I had with her before she passed.

She is gone, and I still fuss over her mindset on a regular basis, for leaving me when we were just getting to the good part. She didn't die due to complications with her diabetes. For that I am thankful. I am proud! I am proud of myself because I helped open her mind and shift her perspective on diabetes management. Together, my aunt and I slowly but surely turned things around. It didn't take fancy tricks or a tremendous amount of effort.

One day as I was thinking about my aunt, I started thinking about all the other people I know and have yet to meet who could benefit from the same help; other people needed the same compassion, understanding, support and encouragement. My therapeutic training and diabetes experience allowed me to have a different type of conversation with my aunt. One that she had not discussed with anyone else. She started reading labels and trying to count carbs. Suddenly, things didn't seem as overwhelming for her. She called me if she was eating something without labels, and we would discuss how many carbs were likely to be in her meal. She started taking her insulin, needles, and glucometer with her when she left the house. I know that sounds crazy, but she was full of shenanigans. My aunt would take her meter without any strips or have the strips and insulin, but no needles. It was always something with her. We took baby steps. They were probably more like little half steps until we built up her courage and know how. Eventually, she got there.

My aunt and I had many serious conversations to get down to the truth of the matter. Tough love and no coddling. These sessions were necessary because she needed to acknowledge what was holding her back. She needed to tell the truth. It all came down to the fact that she was 65, with a plethora of health issues. She thought, "Why should I avoid eating what I love when I'm going to die anyway?" This realization was huge! I was speechless.

I had to take a step back and ask myself, "Why should she do this?" After scratching my head for a second, I said, "While we both know your health is not good, we don't know when your last day will come. Right now you are here, and I want you here as long as you can be." I went on to say, "If you want me to help you, I will because I believe you are worth saving." That was the start of a new beginning for my aunt and me.

From that point on, I decided that it was senseless for another person to hand their life over to diabetes. I was tired of hearing the dialysis stories from my nurse friends. I don't want to hear about another lost limb. I decided to focus my business on helping people with diabetes who feel they are at the end of their rope, people who are tired of fumbling around in the dark with illness. I want to help people open their minds and reignite their passion for better diabetes self-care.

Although I had decided to pursue this path, I wasn't sure if any other people with diabetes might be interested. I wasn't sure I could help anyone else. Then I had a meeting with one of my favorite people. She was once my professor and surrogate mother while I was in college. She taught me much more than the Child and Family Development courses listed in her syllabus. Over the years, we kept in touch, and on this occasion, I went to visit her at work. We had been talking about life, love, and happiness when I mentioned that my son had type 1 diabetes. She told me she had type 2 and acknowledged how terrible it was. I shared with her my thoughts about the senselessness of the condition and how problems could be avoided by doing a few things differently. Initially, she thought she was doing all that she could do to manage her diabetes. For her, that was that.

I did not challenge her. I shared my thoughts on how I wanted to help other people. I had no intention of winning her over. Before I knew it, she was on board. She wanted to know where to sign up! I was elated. I was shocked because she had been so sure of her approach. She said she was doing the best she could, but now she was open to making a few changes. This was a turning point because I wasn't asking and I didn't see it coming.

I am a woman of faith, and I believe that everything happens for a reason. I am beginning to see how we might have won the diabetes lotto (although I'm still waiting on my 20 million). While we continue searching for a cure, I want to be about the business of reigniting the flame in others. I want to help people unlock their minds, guide them to accept their diagnosis and change how they manage diabetes so that they can add healthier years to their lives.

Here is why I said in the beginning that this book is not for everyone. It is for those who have read it all, tried it all and are ready to get off the hamster wheel of symptoms and consequences. This book is for diabetes veterans (long time suffers) dealing with burnout.

If you have low or near perfect A1C's, if you have a healthy meal plan and if you exercise regularly, you might not find much value in what I have to say. You may already know it all. However, this book might be a good resource for your friends and relatives with diabetes who are not managing as well as you are. I wrote this book because I am tired of people without diabetes telling people with diabetes what they should and shouldn't be doing. For the few people without diabetes who do have knowledge on the subject, I want to give you a different perspective on how to help your friends and relatives. You can help them connect with the reality of their situation and jumpstart their reengagement with diabetes self-management.

To work with me, I always tell people that I have two requirements. You must tell the truth, and you must do your work. I cannot do this for you, no one can, but I will help you. I will be by your side without judgment. I will walk you through the necessary steps to shift your perspective for better diabetes management.

Right now, it's just you and me. Let's take our shoes off, get in a comfy position and just get real. No jokes. There is no need to hide, no need to lie, and no need to twist the truth. The truth is your truth, and we will start with that. The fact that you found this book, picked it up, flipped through the pages and then actually bought it, means you or someone you know needs to do better. You want to feel better. You deserve better. And because you have purchased this book, we are family! You invited me in, and now I am here with you. You were searching for something; you found me and the good news is, I want to help you.

I believe you deserve to live! Not exist, not get by, not take one day at a time, but live a full, healthy, happy life. For you to do this, you should feel uncomfortable as you stand in your truth and admit things you usually keep bottled up. This is only making things harder for you. After it is all said and done, you will feel better. You will look better and move around easier. You will be equipped with the tools you need to have more productive conversations with your family and healthcare providers.

CHAPTER TWO

Acceptance vs. Denial

How much are you willing to pay to avoid your condition? What are the consequences? Are they worth it? I get it; you are tired. What is the point anyway? "Life is short, so I may as well eat what I want." Right? Something else I have heard is, "Why change what I eat when I could die tomorrow?" Let's explore a few reasons why you should fight for your life.

1. Your diagnosis is not your fault.

2. From day one, you were never set up to succeed.

3. You don't know what you don't know.

Some people with diabetes never got off to a good start. It is not your fault. Were you ever taught how to manage your condition? Did you ever have your diabetes educator on speed dial for every question you had? If you did, did you feel stupid for needing to call so often? Did you ever sit down with a nutritionist and discuss what your absolute favorite foods were? Did you ever talk and create a plan on what to modify and what to eliminate?

If you did, kudos. If you did not, you are not alone. I have spoken to a lot of people who never had these opportunities. There were times when I expected more of my healthcare team than they were trained to provide. I didn't know what I didn't know. This way of thinking led to unrealistic expectations. When we visit our health care providers, they often want to treat us from their medical or pharmaceutical model. They act as if their only job is to manage the medicine. It seems like all they want to do is throw a pill at the problem. Or cut the problem out of you. It sometimes seems as if a conversation about your emotional state or diet is not important to them. They act as if an investigation into your diet is for someone else to discuss. It is the nutritionist or the diabetes educator's job, right?

Our endocrinologist manages everything diabetes related. They monitor our son for signs of other autoimmune diseases, but mostly they manage his insulin doses. I have liked my "endo" doctors, but I have expected more of them than they could provide in the past. Several times I asked for tips on how to improve our son's levels with his diet. On three separate occasions, I received the response, "Eat more complex carbs than simple carbs." My only response was a blank stare.

I am a college educated woman, and I had to Google "complex carb breakfast ideas" because I needed to know what a darn complex carb was. Can I get a pamphlet, a PDF link or something?

If we don't accept where we are in our journey, in our truth, we will continue to make poor choices. I did not know as much as I thought about healthy eating. One might say this is obvious given that I am currently overweight. I initially gained weight in college. However, I gained most of my weight after having children. Like many moms, I have tried lots of methods to lose weight over the years. There have been some wins and some losses in regard to permanent weight loss. Therefore, I have learned a ton about healthy eating and meal planning. But there are a lot of other factors to consider when planning meals for a person with diabetes. For instance, I need to consider his starting blood sugar, the time of day, his level of activity, and not just the carb count, but how his body responds to a particular food. There are even more factors. I had to learn all this and more in bits and pieces, one mistake and one high blood sugar reading at a time. I was waiting for the doctors to solve my problems and give me guidance on meal planning, instead of being proactive and researching it for myself.

What does it mean to accept diabetes?

First, let us talk about what it does not mean. It does not mean you will ever enjoy having diabetes. It is not to say you should like the fact that your pancreas or cells are not functioning as they should. It means you will stop treating diabetes like the ugly little stepchild who follows you around, nagging you wherever you go. In time, you will start to see diabetes as the little white angel hanging over your right shoulder asking, "Are you sure you want to eat that?" or, "Is now a good time to eat that?"

To be honest, most days I feel like diabetes is bullying me. Bullies taunt you and pester you until they get what they want. You know how on all the movies they show the big burly kid in the neighborhood who scares all the smaller kids? He takes their lunch money, bicycles, new toys, anything he wants. He is the one stuffing smaller kids into lockers just for fun.

There was a time when I felt like I was the kid being stuffed into a locker. Diabetes is always bossing me around! It dictates what we can eat, how much we can eat, what time of day we eat, if we go out or stay in and eat. It is exhausting!! When our son wakes up, it is like diabetes is saying, "You better check his numbers... or else!" With my chest pumped and head bobbing from side to side, I say, "Or else what?" Diabetes says, "Or else he will be at 400 before you know it and higher later. When you are in the emergency room looking like a bad parent, you will regret it!" I ponder for a second, my chest deflates, my chin drops to my chest, and I commence to checking his blood. I just got bullied by diabetes.

Have you ever been bullied by diabetes? It happens to me all the time! When I am about to fall asleep after a grueling day, I hear diabetes saying, "Don't you think you should check him again? Are you sure he is good for the night? Are you sure? Would you bet his life on it?" In total exasperation, throwing the covers off my body, I'm off to test one last time. Except, once I get back to my warm, cozy bed, I close my eyes only for them to pop back open as I realize… I can't go back to sleep! I'm awake two more hours. Diabetes is a bully!

When our son got his first pump, we were excited, but skeptical. His pump is stocked with all types of alarms and chimes. It's smart and shiny. But it didn't take long before our son started hating it. He hated the alarms that beeped every time something needed to happen. Every time it would go off, in total frustration, he would yell, "What is it now?!" He would fuss about it as if it were an annoying little brother. "It's always beeping and telling me to do something. I am so tired of this beep! Why can't it just be quiet?" It was hilarious, yet not funny at all. He was serious. He was annoyed that his annoying little brother was following him around all day long. As much as the device is a life saver, it's also a snitch (in a good way). We need the valuable information it offers, but give it a rest already! Pumps track everything, the good, the bad and the in between. There is no hiding from it. So now my favorite saying is, "Diabetes is a bully and pumps are snitches, but in a good way." I wear my shirt every day, and you should get one, too!

For me to get out of my bed in the middle of the night to test his blood, sometimes three or four times, I must accept his diabetes! By accepting that my son has diabetes, I am acknowledging that there are things I must do to keep him alive, whether I want to or not. By accepting his diagnosis, there are things we cannot do anymore as a family, like eating a Chocolate Fudge Molten cake at 8 in the evening. If we do, no amount of insulin that will keep the chocolate spike at bay. I now have a love/hate relationship with chocolate. I love it for myself, but I hate it for him. The reality is, if I am in denial, it would be easier to ignore the queues to do what will keep him healthy. It would be simpler to act as if we don't have to count carbs or take his backpack of supplies everywhere we go. It would be easier for you to avoid what you need to do to stay healthy. Denial will make it easier for you to pretend your life is still the same.

Action Item

What does accepting diabetes mean to you?

What will change when you have accepted your diabetes?

How will you give up your anger or fear?

How would it feel no longer being able to simply "not know" how to manage your diabetes?

What excuses must you let go of?

What will it look like once you have accepted your diagnosis? How will others notice the change in you?

CHAPTER THREE

The Need to Grieve

I know the word "grief" seems serious and dark. You might be wondering, "Who died and why do I need to grieve?" That's a fair question. The reason you should consider grieving is that it is likely you never have. For a lot of people, a diabetes diagnosis feels like a death sentence. It is like you are just waiting for all the big bad complications to overtake your life slowly. It feels like your life as you once knew it is over. It feels that way because it is the truth.

I don't mean to sound like a Debbie Downer, but a lot changes for people after diagnosis. This is the place where many people get stuck because they will not grieve to let go of their old life. Imagine if you could no longer walk into the dining room, sit down and eat until your heart and stomach are content. Never mind the fact that dessert has changed or is obsolete. Most of us are not eating mixed fruit with a dollop of whipped cream for dessert. We are eating candy, brownies, cookies, cake, donuts, ice cream. Shall I go on? I think we are on the same page and likely, in the same darn boat.

In your new life, you are starving. You had a low carb breakfast, and a decent lunch, but you ate at 11:30 this morning. On your way home from work you ran a few errands. You bought chips, ice cream, and cookies even though you knew you had no business shopping while you were hungry. On the drive home, you are calculating in your head how long it is going to take to test your blood and cook your meal so that you can time your insulin dosage just right. If you do it the right way, you should take your shot at least 15 minutes before you begin eating. Do you know how long 15 minutes is when your stomach is turning flips and churning like a ball of fire? It's long! You manage not to eat any of the food as you cook it because you don't want to throw off your numbers, but you are about to burst. That garlic bread is almost ready, and it's about to be demolished.

In your old life, you could walk into the kitchen and throw whatever you found in your mouth without hesitation. Your pancreas had your back. No worries. No overnight highs. Those were the good old days. My son is only 10, and I am dreading his eventual change in appetite. When we go out, he already tells waiters that his stomach holds "a lot of food" as he pats it in a circle motion (hilarious)! What am I going to do?

In high school, my best friend and I would come home famished. We would stand in the refrigerator eating fruit, lunch meat, cereal, chips, whatever we could find. We didn't stop until we hit our sweet spot. I am dreading this day for him.

I do give him carb-free snacks, but he doesn't want to eat that all the time. I am teaching him the difference between healthy versus non-healthy foods, but we still like what we like. I would be kidding myself if I planned on him only eating zero-carb snacks for the rest of his life. I am not saying it isn't possible, but I am realistic. And the truth is, I won't always be there to police him. Who is policing you? Who is holding you accountable? Who is supporting you and loving you through the tough moments? All I know is that the process is even more difficult for an adult who does not have anyone to hold them accountable.

It is tough accepting the changes required for your new life, but I believe you deserve to live. I know you can do it. Least of all, if you want to maintain good control of your diabetes, you cannot act as if nothing has changed. Everything has changed!

Just let that sink in. Let your heart hurt if it needs to. Just be still with this thought.

If I were with you in person, I would offer you a big hug. This is real, but you can do it!

Your new life requires that you stick your sensitive fingertips multiple times a day. You have to take pills every day. You have to take shots to keep yourself alive. This is not a matter of vanity. It's not a weight loss shot you are taking to get slim.

You do not get to decide if you have diabetes today. If you do not start taking this process seriously, you may die slowly or quickly, but most certainly you will die sooner than you should have. I know this is getting heavy, but don't jump ship just yet. Children, men, and women have died in their sleep due to this condition. I need this to stop. You deserve to live! Therefore, you must grieve the losses because they are real. There are many, and they are different for each of us. It is unfair, uncool and inconvenient, but necessary.

You should spend every moment of every day trying to keep yourself alive. Thinking about death day in and day out is depressing. So, what do most of us do? We act like nothing has changed. We keep doing the things we used to so we can feel normal! Every time I say the word "normal," imagine yourself wearing a white t-shirt with big bold letters that say "I'm normal!" Being normal is all my son wishes for, that's how I know it's a problem. People with diabetes tell me all the time, "I am allowed to be me." The truth is you cannot make the same choices as the old you. You can no longer eat a bag of chips without reading the label, checking carbs, testing your levels and taking insulin. You can no longer go to Saturday morning brunch and eat your favorite waffle, pancakes, French toast, hash browns and orange juice, then top it with warm maple syrup. It's all carbs! It all breaks down in the body as sugar. Although the meat is protein, it is high in fat which can contribute to higher blood sugars as well. It's an all-around bad deal.

You deserve to grieve the loss of spontaneity and variety. I am not saying you cannot create a new kind of variety, but I know you will miss your old one. Your old life felt warm and fuzzy like your favorite old sweatshirt. This new life feels like a tight t-shirt with a crew neck that is two sizes too small. We won't even get started with how incredibly expensive diabetes management is for most and how extremely lonely it can be at times. I just want you to know that you deserve to grieve. You need to grieve in your own way as a means of acceptance to help you transition. I'm not saying these things to try to scare you straight. It is a big deal! It is your life, and it is different now. It is not just about the carbs, pricking and sticking. It's about everything you must do just to survive another day. A person with diabetes will do more by noon than most people do all day just trying to stay alive. This is not easy.

Action Item

What would grieving look like for you?

Write down a list of things you miss about your old life.

What things do you resent about the new life?

What should you come to terms with to be in control of your

diabetes?

CHAPTER FOUR

Motivation vs. "I Don't Wanna's"

This subject is near and dear to my heart because we must find a way to get motivated and stay motivated every single day. There are so many things I don't want to do every day. I do not want to count carbs. I do not want to measure or portion anything. I don't want to have a mini heart attack when I realize we left home without his supplies. I don't want to force myself to stay awake for four more hours to see how the last set of insulin units are going to affect him. Will it make him low or will he need more units because he is still too high? The list of tasks I don't want to do is as high as

Mount Everest.

Some days my son wakes up ready to go. He will grab his glucose meter and test his blood right away. Other times, he will wake up at 7:00 am but will try to wait until 10:30 am to test. He tries his best to avoid adhering to a schedule. He wants to feel normal! I get it because, before his diagnosis, we could do whatever we wanted to do. We woke up late and ate whatever we wanted without stress. If we went out to dinner and it ran past 7 pm, we could still have dessert. He could eat lunch and still have the birthday cupcakes without worry and planning.

How do we keep our motivation up? My motivation comes from wanting my son to live. I want him to live a good life. I want him to know how to manage his condition, whether he is with us or not. I do not want him to subject himself to all the negatives consequences of diabetes prematurely. Contrary to what I thought, it is not a requirement! It is not inevitable to have kidney failure, amputations, blindness, heart attacks, and strokes. Crazy, right? I thought it was just a matter of time before all the terrible stuff happened. Some people can get rid of their diabetes with enough commitment. The real question is, what will it take for you to commit to life? What is important in your life? What makes you want to be here? Who do you want to be here for? God created you as a one of a kind gift. What gifts are you supposed to share with the world that may not get shared if you die too soon? Do not choose death. Choose life and live well.

I want to take a moment to check on you. How are you? Are you still with me? This is a lot to take in, but you are a fighter. You are courageous, and I know you can do this.

Some people might take issue with the phrase, "Don't choose death." I can hear people saying, "I didn't choose to have diabetes!" You are right. You did not choose to have diabetes, but you do choose how well you take care of yourself. Ignoring your condition and making unhealthy choices are examples of choosing death. I say this with love because we sometimes do not see the reality of our actions. This is heavy. You may even shut this book right now and toss it in the trash. I would rather risk being ridiculed than lie or sugarcoat the truth. Choose life!

I have shared what motivates me. Now I want to know, what will motivate you? When my aunt told me, "What's the point in eating what the doctors want if I'm just going to die anyway?", I was stunned. For a few seconds, I had no rebuttal. She was 65 with a string of health issues. She had a point. It soon became clear, although her health was not great, she was still alive. She was still here with me, fighting the fight and trying to get it right. I wanted more time with her, which is why I wanted her to do her best to live. It almost sounds selfish, but she had other reasons to live. For one, her grandchildren. She loved them with her whole heart. She would do anything for them. I know she would have given her last just to get one more day with them.

I challenge you to uncover your motivations.

Action Item

When you wake up in the morning, what makes you want to live another day?

What is on your "I-don't-wanna" list? Is there anything you can delegate to a friend or loved one who supports you?

What mechanisms can you put in place to help ward off the "I-don't-wanna's?"

Who would be impacted by your absence in this world?

CHAPTER FIVE

Forgiving Yourself

Forgiveness is one of my favorite "F" words. Forgiveness is the gift that keeps on giving in diabetes management. No matter how hard we try, this is never going to be a perfect process. We are not always going to get everything right. We might not test blood sugars when we are supposed to. We may not adequately cover the food we eat, even when we try our best. We may eat a meal loaded with carbs knowing it is not the best choice to make. We are not always going to eat what we should because that peach cobbler with vanilla ice cream just before you pulled the covers over your head was everything", wasn't it? That pecan, pumpkin, apple pie or brownie a la mode was everything! That sweet tooth is real!

We must be honest with ourselves. If tweaking as we go is necessary, that is what we will do. A1C's won't always be where we prefer. Someone reading this book might have an A1C over 13, over 15 or possibly higher. No judgment, just truth. This process is not easy, and it is harder when we hold on to every misstep we make.

Have you ever started the day out saying, "Today is going to be a better day. I am going to eat right, test my blood on time and take my shots correctly"? You wake up feeling good considering the alternatives (headaches, dizziness, etc.). Today you start out strong, while in the back of your mind you recall all the missteps from yesterday. Yesterday, the office catered lunch, and there was no way you were going to miss out on that good free food. Today, you woke up motivated to do better than yesterday. You tested your blood sugar before your toes could hit the floor. It was a little elevated thanks to that peach cobbler. You confirmed your correction instead of just guessing. You gave yourself your shot or took your pills.

To prove how much you were on your game, you ate a healthy breakfast. The real kind, with egg whites, veggies, grapefruit and a piece of toast with almond butter. You didn't even cook your eggs with butter. If you love butter as much as my mother does, this part is not easy. About four hours go by, and you are ready for lunch. Again, you say to yourself, "I am going to do right. You make a chicken and veggie bowl like the one the restaurants make. You make cilantro rice, grilled chicken, grilled bell peppers and onions, beans, tomatoes, homemade guacamole, and load it with sour cream, cheese, and salsa. Talk about good eats.

The health experts are saying, "This meal is not healthy", but it is better than a pizza. We're talking about how people eat, not what they say they eat.

Once more, you grab your glucose meter and pop open the expensive bottle of strips just right to avoid a test strip confetti party! I have been there and almost died looking at all my money on the filthy ground.

Once you have positioned the strip just right and the meter is reading as ready, you grab the lancet and push a button or two. You look at those fingertips and decide which one wins the red dot lotto. You poke and squeeze the finger tightly to get a good drop of blood. Heaven forbid you do not get enough blood on the strip, cause an "error," having to use another expensive strip and poke another finger! You didn't want to poke the first finger! You have neither money, nerves, nor strips to waste.

After avoiding a few small catastrophes, you unconsciously stop breathing as you wait the few seconds to find out whether you get a high five for getting it right or if you need Botox to fill those frown lines between your eyes from trying to figure out how you went wrong. "Ding!" The verdict is in, and you get a high five! You did it! You got it right. With blood sugars in range, you can feel even better about eating the lunch you made. You administer your insulin and take the first bite.

Four hours later, it's time for dinner. You are excited. You feel good about redeeming yourself after yesterday's feast. You feel so good that you start planning a treat for dessert. You go through your ritual of pulling out the glucose meter, popping the strips open just right, pricking and squeezing your finger, ending up with the perfect droplet. You got it onto the strip without error. This time you are feeling good about yourself, so you take a few shallow breaths while you wait for the results. Evidence of your effort is on the line. This is your blood, sweat, and tears, trying to be on target for both breakfast and lunch. "Ding!" The verdict is in. 389? "How am I at 389? I made a healthy lunch!", you think to yourself.

You are so baffled that you run through your previous meals trying to figure out what went wrong. Do you know what went wrong? Write in the margin if you do. As you look at everything you put in the veggie and chicken bowl, you question whether you over did it with the rice. You did have a pretty big helping of sour cream. The truth is, you forgot to measure your rice. You decided last minute to eyeball it. You are frustrated. You always try to measure food on days you are "eating right."

Suddenly, it dawns on you that you are usually high after that meal, but you decided that it was not a big deal because it's one of your favorite meals and it "was worth it." Today, it doesn't feel good. You are disappointed that you worked hard all day to keep your numbers good and now you are high. You take a deep breath, drop your shoulders and sit there. You think, "I am already high, so I should just eat what I want and try to cover it." Next, you think, "Maybe I should just continue my path because I was doing so well today." You take a few more seconds and think about it. Finally, you say "Nah!" and commence to eating your dinner with dessert. This time you guess at your sliding scale and hope your insulin coverage will be enough.

Am I making this up or have you or a loved one been here before? If you have, it is okay. It is normal. This is real life for many people with diabetes. Sometimes we know we are making a poor choice and other times we don't know until our numbers slap us across the face. It is so easy to get discouraged. And it is even easier to stay there. Take baby steps and think about what it would be like to let go of all the missteps you are holding on to. Figure out what the miscalculation was, make a note for future reference and <u>move on</u>. Forgive yourself and forget the error. Do not hold on to the times when things did no go right. You need all your energy to help you stay focused on moving forward and doing well tomorrow, the next day and the day after that. Give yourself a thousand do-overs. Live in the present, not the past!

Action Item

What would it feel like to let go of all your failures?

How would your life be different if you let go of the missteps?

How would people be able to tell by looking at you or talking to you?

List at least one misstep you could work on letting go of. List more if you like.

CHAPTER SIX

Honesty in Diabetes

"To thine own self be true!" In all things, we must be honest with ourselves. I did not say we must be honest with other people." At some point in our lives, we have lied to someone. When you think back on lies you have told, how much did the lie help your relationship with that person? Maybe it kept you out of trouble for a moment, but what kind of relationship is it if you must lie? I will never forget living on a Navy base in Meridian, Mississippi with my mom and stepdad at the time. I recall the day my mom and I went to wash clothes at the laundromat. It was a gray building with a small convenience store attached to the side.

After loading the washers, my mom and I went to the store to get something she had forgotten at home. As she looked around, I was where every child would be, the candy isle. They had these little orange candies in a miniature orange juice carton. I thought it was just too cute. I had to have it. It was so tiny. It was just the right size for my little hand. Up until that point, I had never seen such a small carton. I was amazed by it.

I can remember my Mom giving me "the speech" before we went in. The one that starts with, "Don't you ask for nothing in this store…" and goes on with a few more threats, which she was happy to act on if necessary. I couldn't ask her to buy it for me, so I decided to take it. She paid for her things and, at some point, I slid the cute little OJ carton into my pocket. We went back to check on the clothes. I was so happy that I had my cute little OJ carton. I analyzed the carton, wondering what the candy would taste like. As I started trying to figure out how I was going to eat the candy without being noticed, my heart started racing and my breathing sped up. I started getting nervous.

I realized there was no way I was going to eat this candy without my mother seeing me. I wouldn't be able to eat it in front of her because she knew I didn't have any money. What lie was going to get me through this one? I couldn't lie and say I got it from a friend. If I couldn't eat the candy, what was it all for? I was about to get the beating of the century for nothing. This was devastating. Just as I was about to put it back into my pocket, she caught me. I was so scared. I immediately felt shame and sheer terror. My mother is a fusser and a yeller. She took me back to the store immediately. Luckily, I had not opened it yet, so she made me give the candy back to the owner. I had to look the store owner in the face and apologize. I was so embarrassed. I could not believe she was making me do this. I knew what I had done wrong, but this was humiliating.

Those were simpler times. No cops were involved. The store owner didn't even make her pay for it; he just took it back. I could tell he understood. He was on her side. He could tell this wasn't the end of her wrath. She was just getting started. Back then parents had each other's back, so he knew she was going to handle things. Of course, that spanking was coming when I got home. It was the worst day ever. I learned two things that day: never lie and never steal. Growing up, we were always told, "If you lie, you'll steal" and neither are worth the consequences.

When you lie, you have to look over your shoulder. You are worried whether you will be found out or not. You worry about what people will think of you because of the lie. You are stressed out and cannot be at peace with yourself. You can't truly be proud of yourself. How can you live with integrity when you are always lying? It isn't in our nature to lie. As adults, we know right from wrong. We know lying does not produce anything good. The question is, "What happens when we lie to ourselves?" It is ten times worse because you already know the truth. Therefore, you are not fooling anybody.

Lies will keep you from seeing people and situations as they truly are. If we lie to ourselves long enough, we start believing them. Here is where things get dangerous. Lying to yourself can cause you to end up in situations you have no business in. It can distort your sense of reality. As it relates to diabetes, it can cause you to act like you do not have diabetes when you know you do.

The distorted reality will have you believe the things you are eating are not that bad most of the time. It will lead you to believe that it is okay only to test your blood sugar after your vision has gone blurry and you cannot stop downing glasses of water.

The lies will make you feel like sporadically taking your pills is okay. Not a big deal, right? I didn't take my pill this morning, but I can eat this cinnamon roll with sweetened coffee". It's not a big deal to skip a pill, right? All lies! Deadly lies. No one wants to think about the end game of diabetes, but too many people have left this world due to complications from mismanagement, or non-management, of their diabetes.

Is death worth it?

Some people live a long, terrible, unhealthy life with diabetes and don't die right away. However, their bodies are deteriorating slowly, day by day. They go blind.

They lose toes, feet, and legs. Their internal organs start shutting down. Dialysis is a beast not to be played with. Someone reading this book is already facing what I just described. Others are on their way. My goal is to stop you. There is light and life on the other side of this situation.

You deserve to live. You deserve to feel better. You deserve a long life. However, you must choose it. Despite all the sugar and salt in American food, you must choose it. Your favorite foods will always be there. Your love for them is likely never to change, but if you decide to change how you think about your life, it will help you create a level of control you have never exercised before.

There is no magic pill, for many, there is no cure, and it will never be easy. However, it can be done if you get honest with yourself. Be honest about what is not working when it comes to your diabetes management. People are at various stages, so it is important to figure out what your struggles are. Is it acceptance? Have you accepted the diagnosis, but it is too much to manage with all the other things going on in your life? Do you manage a little here and there, but there is no consistency? Do you know what diabetes is and what you should be doing? Do you leave your doctor appointments feeling like you understood what was said? Or do you feel like everything they said went straight over your head?

Have you accepted your diagnosis and tried to do what you are supposed to, but you feel lonely because the people in your life just do not understand? Friends might keep inviting you out to places that trigger you to eat all the things you should avoid. Do you have know-it-all relatives who want to tell you what you should and should not be eating?

Do you find yourself rebelling from

the regimen and just wish to be normal again for one day? One day without thinking about food and carbs. One day without timing everything just right. No finger sticks, no injections, no tubing, no bag full of medical supplies and snacks.

Be honest and tell your truth! It's okay; this is a safe place. Just be yourself and stay true to you.

Action Item

Make a list of things you need to be honest about.

Circle the top 5 most important ones that are keeping you stuck in a rut.

How would your life be different if you were honest about your condition?

CHAPTER SEVEN

Patience is a Virtue

Be as patient with yourself as you would a two-day old baby. Patience can be a difficult thing for some people, but to start fresh with a blank slate every day, you must learn to be patient with yourself.

After realizing my denial and accepting that diabetes was going to be part of our lives, I grieved the loss of the life we once lived; I grieved the loss of convenience, flexibility, and spontaneity. I had to get honest about what was working and what was not. As a parent of a child with type 1, my choices are a huge part of a high A1C number. We attributed it to several different situations, but after a three-month period of highs, I knew I was doing something wrong. To be clear, my endocrinologist didn't call us out. She just adjusted the numbers and told us to limit the "simple carbs", which I did not fully understand at the time.

I had to forgive myself for not doing better and for not getting it right every day. I had to find ways to stay motivated each day. I had to stay vigilant and on top of diabetes. This forgiveness led me to patience. Anyone who knows me knows patience has never been my thing. I am in a hurry to finish typing this darn sentence! I hate patience. When it comes to working on myself, I am not patient. My negative self-talk says, "I should already have this down." The truth is, even if I do have it down, things frequently change in diabetes management. Not to mention the fact that it is ten times harder to manage diabetes for someone else. Are there any parents or caregivers out there who can relate?

If it were me, I could buckle down and say "no" to certain foods. I could negotiate with myself about things. In my case, I am helping and teaching my son, who is a growing, hungry boy. I love our endocrinologist, but she keeps telling me to give him fewer simple carbs and to swap those with more complex carbs. Did I lose anyone? She means to feed my son more carbs from veggies and whole fruit instead of bread, pasta, and rice. That is easier said than done. My son takes after my mom, and he loves bread. Therefore, we have lots of disagreements about food. What to eat, when to eat, how much to eat, how much more to eat. It just never ends. I need lots of patience to help see through all these little daily battles.

Exercising patience keeps me from sweating the small stuff and the big stuff. Even if we make a big "oops," all we can do is discuss what happened, identify the error, make a note and create a new plan for next time. We can give a snack or a shot, treat the high or low and move on to the next issue in diabetes for the day. There are more to come, so move on. If you keep holding on, it will start to weigh on your confidence. Often this only causes you to make more poor choices. You will think, "Oh well, I'm messing up anyway." Do not fall for this.

People with diabetes do not hear enough, "You are doing the best you can! You are doing a good job!" If you are not doing a good job and you are not doing the best you can do, do better. Today is a new day. Ask for what you need. If you need more help than what was provided during the initial hospital stay, ask! Demand that your doctors help you. That is what we pay them for. Most importantly give yourself a break. Small steps can create big changes.

ACTION ITEM

What does patience look and feel like to you?

How would your life be different if you were patient with yourself?

What would it be like if, after a high, you gently patted yourself on the back and said, "It will be okay. Let's fix it?"

List the three reasons why it is difficult being patient with yourself.

CHAPTER EIGHT

Your Healthcare Team

In the months after the diagnosis, my son's A1C was great. We were on bottles and needles, but they were killing me. It became stressful because it seemed like we were always dealing with either very high or very low numbers. Trying to find a middle ground felt impossible. There was a period when we got the home numbers under control, but we started having communication issues with the school nurse. He would be high during school hours for days, and I would be unaware because the temporary nurse refused to use a computer to send me his numbers.

After visiting the endocrinologist every three months, I found myself trying all kinds of things to solve the problem. I felt terrible that I was not doing better. I started feeling like I needed a shirt that read, "I'm doing the best I can!" I felt like, no matter what reasons I found for the highs, our endo knew the problem was in the diet, even though she never said it. My guilt got to the point where I started asking my husband to take our son to the endocrinology visits instead of me. My husband is built differently than I am. He doesn't let things affect him the way I do, so I started sending him.

More time passed, and we still were not seeing any significant improvements despite our regular doctor's visits. I love my endo. She is sweet and smart. She never comes off as judgmental. She does all the things good endos do. She looks at his patterns and numbers. She chats with my son; she does his mini-physical and finally makes the necessary adjustments to his doses. Still, I just was not satisfied with his numbers. I decided something needed to change. I started asking her about his diet. I told her what he was eating and where we were running into problems. Again, I heard, "You would want to limit the simple carbs and increase complex carbs." There was a point where I thought he was eating enough complex carbs. I was too embarrassed to admit that I didn't have a clue. Diabetes has so many moving parts that it took a long time to isolate the problem and figure out where we were going wrong.

We visited my son's pediatrician who performed his "well child checkup." She would ask how things were going with his diabetes, but since it was not her specialty, not much was offered in the way of solutions. Looking back, I see I was waiting for the doctors to give me more direction, but that never happened. In my mind, it made total sense for them to tell us the specific dietary changes to make. They would complete the screenings, adjust his doses and send us on our way.

I thought I was making decent choices with meal planning, but the A1C was showing us otherwise. It was 8 when they wanted it at 6-7. After a few rounds of this, I finally started to realize there was a problem. It was me. I thought about all the times I caved in and let him have something when I knew he shouldn't. I recalled the times where we got home after 7 pm, and I had to serve dinner late. It sounds strange, but we needed to have enough time for him to eat dinner, followed by a few hours to digest before bedtime. We had to retest his blood sugar before bed and sometimes give my son a snack to prevent overnight lows. There were not enough hours in the day!

I try to make things as fair as I can when I can and sometimes it gets me into trouble. Simply sharing a dessert at dinner can lead to late night highs, causing me to be up until 5 am when I work at 8 am! Additionally, I did not understand the impact of my son's simple carb breakfasts. He would have two mini sausage breakfast sandwiches (26 carbs), ½ cup unsweetened apple (13 carbs) and 4 ounces of orange juice (14 carbs), totaling 53 of his allowed 60 carbs per meal. From my point of view, we were good. We weren't even at 60 carbs (as directed by his doctor)!

We didn't figure out the impact of his breakfast until we bought our Dexcom Continuous Glucose Monitor. It has been a saving grace. We soon learned that carbs were the problem. As soon as we lowered his carbs things were easier to manage, and his numbers went down. We had been fumbling in the dark until the Dexcom brought us into the light.

I figured out on my own that the night time snacks were messing us up. Even after he changed to insulin pens, I decided midday snacks needed to go. There were times when our endo was hesitant to go with my plan, but I was tired, and something had to change. I was learning the hard way that I was my son's best advocate. I had to figure out the hard way that when I stepped into a doctor's office, it wasn't a sit and listen session. I was not a spectator in this healthcare process. This conversation should be a dialogue between two educated individuals who are trying to craft the best plan possible for you.

To be fair, I do not entirely blame the doctors because the state of our healthcare system is larger than them. I believe most doctors are well intentioned. Due to the state of managed care in the U.S., they don't have a lot of time to engage with their patients. The doctors bought into the medical model like the rest of us. However, I do feel it is within their scope to provide resources regarding healthy eating and meal planning for patients. They should ask specific and in-depth questions regarding diet to help decide where we are getting off track. That is the nutritionist's area, you say? Well, get one on staff and while you are at it, get the therapist on staff, as well. We must stop treating illnesses in bite-sized pieces. We must start treating the whole person. People are likely to avoid calling the nutritionist and their therapist until things get bad. We can do better in America. I believe we can.

I no longer sit by waiting for doctors to treat my son holistically. If we come into the office with higher than preferred A1Cs, we need to discuss at length what is happening with our diet and in our lives. Increasing insulin doses is not the best idea when we can eat smarter. I don't expect the doctors to be nutritionists, but better discussions are needed. Some people are fortunate enough to have a doctor who discusses meal planning and nutrition. Not everyone is so lucky. Not everyone knows that they should demand more from their healthcare team.

Today, I wish I had a "Diabetic Nutritionist" on speed dial. I don't know if that exists, but it should. I do know that not all nutritionists are familiar with the specific needs of people with diabetes. I love my diabetes educator because she knows nutrition and diabetes. Unfortunately, she was busy at her hospital; she could not hold our hands for long. However, no matter how much time has passed, she helps us if we need her. We love our diabetes educator but most importantly, do you have one? Stop accepting the diabetes status quo. Stop accepting good enough. Stop accepting mediocre care. Stop being a spectator and become your best advocate.

Action Item

What past medical experiences are preventing you from feeling comfortable with your healthcare team?

What would it look like if you became your own advocate and took control of your healthcare?

What makes you hesitant to have an open and collaborative conversation with your doctors?

How can you better educate yourself on your condition?

CHAPTER NINE

Closing Thoughts

YOU MADE IT!

Making it to the end of this book tells me a lot about you. It tells me you are committed. It tells me that you do care about the state of your health or your loved one's health. We have discussed a lot. I want to thank you for sticking it out with me. Diabetes management is a marathon, not a sprint. We must grieve, forgive ourselves, be honest, stay motivated, have patience, be our own advocate and above all else, accept your diabetes diagnosis.

Be open-minded and know that you are not alone. This process feels like it is something worth giving up because it can be so hard. Know that you are an amazing person. You are wanted on this earth. I don't want anyone to die because of a diagnosis of diabetes that can be controlled. I hear you. I see the pain and the suffering you are going through. I am here for you, and I want you to know that every step you take, I am proud of you. As you go forward in life, I am here to remind you that you can push through.

What do I know? I had to work through each one of these steps to make better choices, correct mistakes and demand the support I needed from my healthcare team. It's time for you to do the same.

If any of the topics discussed resonate with you, and you would like to take a deeper dive into what is holding you back, go to www.ADiabeticLife.com where you can sign up for a free tip sheet to help you remember the key points of this book. You can also hop over to Facebook and join our group: @https://www.facebook.co m/groups/1079662862101360/

I would love for you to join a community of like-minded individuals who are working hard every day to live healthier, happier lives with diabetes. I would love to hear your thoughts about the book - good, bad or indifferent. Feel free to email me:

carmella@adiabetictypelife.com

I am available for Keynote, workshop, and seminar opportunities.

ABOUT THE AUTHOR

Carmella Bell lives in Fresno, Texas with her awesome husband and two of the smartest kids on the planet. In 2012, diabetes snuck into their lives and stole their trust and spontaneity at a moment's notice when her son was diagnosed with type 1 diabetes. At this point, Carmella learned how little her Aunt Carolyn didn't know about her diabetes diagnosis. This information opened Carmella's eyes to the plight of thousands of type 2 diabetics who are struggling. Carmella's 7 Steps to Push Through Diabetes Overwhelm became a reality when she realized the number of people succumbing to the harsh realities of diabetes were never equipped to succeed. Carmella Bell is a Diabetes Strategist, who earned a bachelor's and a master's degree in Psychology. She is a licensed Marriage and Family Therapist Associate and the founder of A Diabetic Type Life Coaching and Consulting Company. Carmella is a natural born advocate who embodies the gift of encouragement. She has motivated, inspired and transformed the lives of others throughout the years with her no-nonsense, yet loving approach to coaching.